LIVING WITH HERPES:

A GUIDE TO MANAGING SYMPTOMS AND STIGMA

BY

DR. CHARLIE DAVE

COPYRIGHT

FOREWARD

"Dear reader, I want you to know that you are not alone. Living with herpes can be a challenging and isolating experience, but it doesn't define your worth or identity. You are more than your diagnosis, and you deserve compassion, understanding, and support.

This book is a safe space for you to explore your feelings, concerns, and hopes. It's a resource to help you navigate the physical and emotional aspects of herpes, and to find empowerment and resilience.

Remember, herpes is a common and manageable condition. You are not shameful or dirty because of it. You are a person deserving of love, care, and respect - from yourself and others.

As you read these pages, know that you are part of a community that understands and cares. We are here to support you, to listen without judgment, and to help you thrive.

With compassion and understanding."

[Charlie Dave]

Catalog

PART ONE: UNDERSTANDING HERPES

INTRODUCTION TO HERPES

Herpes is a common sexually transmitted infection (STI) caused by a group of viruses. It can cause painful blisters or sores on the genitals, mouth, or other areas of the body. While there's no cure for herpes, there are effective treatments to manage outbreaks and reduce transmission risk.

This guide aims to empower you with knowledge about herpes, its different types, transmission, and available resources. It's important to remember:

You're not alone. Herpes is incredibly common, affecting millions of people worldwide.

With proper management, herpes doesn't have to significantly impact your life or relationships.

Open communication with sexual partners is crucial for informed decisions and healthy intimacy.

What is Herpes?

Herpes is caused by a group of viruses belonging to the herpesvirus family. These viruses can remain dormant in nerve cells for extended periods, occasionally reactivating to cause outbreaks characterized by blisters or sores.

TYPES OF HERPES

The two main types of herpes viruses causing STIs are:

Herpes simplex virus type 1 (HSV-1): Primarily associated with oral herpes, causing cold sores around the mouth and lips. However, HSV-1 can also spread to the genitals through oral sex.

Herpes simplex virus type 2 (HSV-2): Primarily responsible for genital herpes, causing blisters or sores on the genitals, buttocks, or thighs.

Types of Herpes and Their Symptoms

Here's a breakdown of the most common types of herpes and their characteristic symptoms:

Oral Herpes (HSV-1):

Symptoms: Clusters of small, fluid-filled blisters around the mouth and lips, often preceded by tingling, itching, or burning sensations.

Transmission: Primarily through oral-to-oral contact, including kissing, sharing utensils, or drinking glasses.

Frequency: Very common, with estimates suggesting a majority of adults carry HSV-1 antibodies.

Severity: Outbreaks may be mild or severe, with the frequency varying significantly between individuals.

Genital Herpes (HSV-2):

Symptoms: Clusters of small, painful blisters or sores on the genitals, buttocks, or thighs. Outbreaks can be accompanied by flu-like symptoms such as fever, fatigue, and swollen lymph nodes during the first infection.

Transmission: Primarily through skin-to-skin contact during vaginal, anal, or oral sex with someone infected with HSV-2. Transmission can occur even when there are no visible sores present (asymptomatic shedding).

Frequency: Approximately 1 in 6 Americans between 14-49 years old have HSV-2.

Severity: Outbreaks may be mild or severe, with the frequency varying between individuals.

Less Common Types:

Varicella-Zoster Virus (VZV): Causes chickenpox and shingles. Can also cause a type of herpes infection in the genital area but is less common than HSV-1 or HSV-2.

Epstein-Barr Virus (EBV): Causes infectious mononucleosis ("mono") and can also cause a type of herpes infection.

HOW IS HERPES TRANSMITTED

Herpes can be transmitted through skin-to-skin contact with an infected person during an outbreak, even when sores are not visible (asymptomatic shedding). The risk of transmission increases with the presence of open sores.

Here are some ways herpes can be spread:

Vaginal, anal, or oral sex: This is the most common way for HSV-2 to spread.

Oral-to-oral contact: This can transmit HSV-1 from the mouth to the genitals (oral herpes) or vice versa.

Sharing personal items: Sharing towels, washcloths, or razors with someone infected with herpes can increase the risk, although this is less common.

Skin-to-skin contact: Touching infected areas (sores) can transmit the virus, though this is less common.

From mother to baby: In rare cases, a pregnant woman with herpes can pass the virus to her baby during childbirth.

It's Important to Note:

You cannot contract herpes from toilet seats, swimming pools, or hot tubs.

Sharing utensils or glasses with someone who has oral herpes is unlikely to cause genital herpes.

Using condoms consistently and correctly can significantly reduce the risk of transmission, but it doesn't eliminate it entirely.

HERPES SYMPTOMS AND DIAGNOSIS

Demystifying Herpes: Symptoms, Diagnosis, and Test Results

Herpes, a common sexually transmitted infection (STI), can feel overwhelming due to the associated stigma and lack of complete understanding. However, with accurate information and guidance, you can effectively navigate diagnosis, treatment, and maintain healthy relationships. This guide explores common symptoms, diagnosis methods, and interpreting test results to empower you with knowledge and address any concerns you might have.

Recognizing the Signs: Common Symptoms of Herpes

Oral Herpes (HSV-1):

Clusters of small, fluid-filled blisters typically around the mouth and lips (cold sores)

Tingling, itching, or burning sensations at the outbreak site before blisters appear

Swollen lymph nodes in the neck

Fever (less common)

Genital Herpes (HSV-2):

Clusters of small, painful blisters or sores on the genitals, buttocks, or thighs

Burning, itching, or tingling sensations in the genital area before sores appear

Pain when urinating

Vaginal discharge (in females)

Swollen lymph nodes in the groin

Flu-like symptoms such as fever, fatigue, and headache (especially during the first infection)

Important Points:

Not everyone with herpes experiences symptoms. Some individuals may have outbreaks so mild they go unnoticed (asymptomatic shedding).

Symptoms can vary from person to person and may decrease in frequency and severity over time.

Other conditions can mimic herpes symptoms, making diagnosis by symptoms alone unreliable.

Seeking Clarity: Diagnosis Methods for Herpes

If you experience symptoms suggestive of herpes, seeking professional medical advice is crucial. Here's what you can expect during a diagnosis process:

Medical History: Your doctor will discuss your medical history, sexual practices, and any current symptoms.

Physical Examination: A visual examination of the genitals or mouth may be conducted to check for sores.

Diagnostic Tests: While a visual exam can raise suspicion, confirmatory tests are needed for accurate diagnosis. Several tests are available:

Viral Culture: A swab sample from a sore is taken and sent to a lab to grow the virus. This test takes several days to produce results but can be highly accurate.

Polymerase Chain Reaction (PCR) Test: This test detects the herpes virus's genetic material in a swab sample. It's fast and highly accurate, but may not differentiate between HSV-1 and HSV-2.

Blood Test: This test detects antibodies your body produces in response to the herpes virus. Blood tests can tell you if you've ever been infected with HSV-1 or HSV-2, but cannot determine if you're currently contagious.

Understanding Your Test Results:

Positive Viral Culture or PCR Test: This confirms the presence of the herpes virus and indicates an active infection.

Negative Viral Culture or PCR Test: A negative test result doesn't necessarily rule out herpes. It's possible the test was done too early in the outbreak or the virus wasn't present in the sampled area.

Positive Blood Test for HSV-1/2: This indicates you've been infected with the virus at some point in your life. However, it doesn't distinguish between HSV-1 and HSV-2, nor does it confirm current infection.

IgG Antibodies: These antibodies typically appear weeks or months after infection and indicate a long-term immune response.

IgM Antibodies: These antibodies appear earlier in the infection but may not always be present. They can suggest a recent infection.

Negative Blood Test for HSV-1/2: This doesn't necessarily mean you haven't been infected. It's possible your body hasn't developed detectable antibodies yet.

Interpreting Your Results with a Healthcare Professional

Test results should always be interpreted in conjunction with your medical history and symptom presentation. Here's why consulting your doctor is crucial:

Understanding the Implications: Your doctor can explain what your results mean in the context of your specific situation. For example, a positive blood test for HSV-2 means you've been infected but doesn't necessarily confirm genital herpes.

Discussing Treatment Options: Depending on the type of herpes and severity of your infection, your doctor can discuss treatment options like antiviral medications to manage outbreaks and reduce transmission risk.

Addressing Future Risks: If you're diagnosed with herpes, your doctor can provide guidance on minimizing transmission to partners and maintaining a healthy sex life.

Remember, You're Not Alone

A diagnosis of herpes can be emotionally challenging. However, it's important to remember:

Herpes is a very common STI. Millions of people worldwide live healthy lives with herpes.

With proper management, herpes doesn't significantly impact your sex life or relationships.

PART 2: MANAGING SYMPTOMS

MEDICATION AND TREATMENT OPTIONS

Receiving a herpes diagnosis can stir up emotions like fear, anxiety, and maybe even shame. However, knowledge is power. This section delves into the world of managing herpes symptoms, offering a clear picture of available medications, treatment options, and even exploring alternative therapies.

The Power of Antivirals: Suppressing and Shortening Outbreaks

Antiviral medications are the mainstay of herpes management. These medications work by interfering with the virus's ability to replicate, preventing outbreaks or shortening their duration and severity. Here's what you need to know:

Types of Antiviral Medications: Acyclovir (Zovirax), Valacyclovir (Valtrex), and Famciclovir (Famvir) are the three main antiviral medications used for treating herpes. They come in tablet form and are typically taken orally.

Episodic Therapy: This approach involves taking medication only when symptoms appear (outbreak therapy). It can shorten the duration and severity of an outbreak but doesn't prevent future outbreaks.

Suppressive Therapy: This approach involves taking medication daily, even when you don't have symptoms. Suppressive therapy can significantly reduce the frequency and severity of outbreaks and also decrease the risk of transmitting the virus to your partner(s) during periods of asymptomatic shedding (when you don't have visible sores).

Important Considerations:

Dosage and Duration: Your doctor will determine the appropriate dosage and duration of your antiviral medication regimen based on the type of herpes, severity of your outbreaks, and your individual needs.

Side Effects: Antiviral medications are generally well-tolerated, but some individuals may experience mild side effects like nausea, headache, or dizziness.

Resistance: While uncommon, prolonged or improper use of antiviral medications can lead to viral resistance. It's crucial to follow your doctor's instructions regarding dosage and duration of treatment.

Beyond Antivirals: Exploring Additional Treatment Options

While antiviral medications are the cornerstone of managing outbreaks, other approaches can be helpful:

Pain Management: During outbreaks, the sores can be painful. Over-the-counter pain relievers like ibuprofen or acetaminophen can help alleviate discomfort. Additionally, applying topical anesthetic creams like lidocaine can numb the area and provide temporary relief.

Sitz Baths: Soaking your genital area in warm water (sitz bath) for 10-15 minutes several times a day can provide soothing relief and promote healing.

Stress Management: Stress can trigger outbreaks. Practicing relaxation techniques like yoga, meditation, or deep breathing can help manage stress and potentially reduce outbreak frequency.

Maintaining a Healthy Lifestyle: A healthy diet, regular exercise, and adequate sleep can strengthen your immune system, making it better equipped to fight off outbreaks.

Exploring Alternative Therapies:

It's important to manage expectations when considering alternative therapies for herpes. While some may offer some relief, there's no scientific evidence to support them as cures. Here are some options you might encounter:

Lysine: This amino acid is a popular alternative therapy for herpes. While studies suggest it may help reduce outbreak frequency, the evidence is inconclusive.

Zinc: Zinc supplementation may shorten the duration of outbreaks, but more research is needed to confirm its effectiveness.

Probiotics: Probiotics may contribute to a healthy immune system, potentially impacting outbreak frequency, but further research is necessary.

Remember:

It's crucial to discuss any alternative therapies with your doctor before trying them. They can help you weigh the potential benefits and risks and ensure they won't interfere with your prescribed medications.

Communication is Key: Partner Management and Reducing Transmission Risk

Having herpes shouldn't prevent you from having healthy, fulfilling relationships. Open and honest communication with potential and existing partners is essential. Here are some tips:

Disclosure: Be upfront and honest about your herpes status with potential partners before engaging in sexual intimacy.

Educate Yourself and Your Partner: Share reliable information about herpes transmission and management with your partner(s).

Safer Sex Practices: Consistent and correct condom use can significantly reduce the risk of transmission, even though it doesn't eliminate it entirely.

Suppressive Therapy: If you're in a committed relationship, talk to your doctor about suppressive therapy. This can significantly lower the risk of transmission to your partner.

LIFESTYLE CHANGES FOR MANAGING SYMPTOMS

While antiviral medications are a mainstay in managing herpes outbreaks, a holistic approach incorporating healthy lifestyle practices can significantly improve your well-being. This section explores how diet, exercise, stress management, sleep hygiene, and self-care can contribute to a stronger immune system, potentially reducing outbreak frequency and severity.

Diet and Nutrition: Fueling Your Body for Optimal Health

What you eat directly impacts your immune system's ability to fight off infections. Here are some dietary strategies to consider:

Balanced Diet: Focus on a well-balanced diet rich in fruits, vegetables, and whole grains. These foods are packed with vitamins, minerals, and antioxidants that support immune function.

Lean Protein Sources: Include lean protein sources like fish, poultry, beans, and lentils in your diet. Protein is essential for building and repairing tissues, which is crucial during outbreaks when your body is healing.

Healthy Fats: Include healthy fats from sources like avocados, nuts, and olive oil in your diet. These fats contribute to a healthy immune response.

Stay Hydrated: Drinking plenty of water throughout the day keeps you hydrated and helps flush out toxins, promoting overall well-being.

Foods to Limit:

Highly Processed Foods: Processed foods are often high in sugar, unhealthy fats, and sodium, which can contribute to inflammation and potentially worsen outbreaks.

Refined Sugars: Sugary foods can cause blood sugar spikes and potentially weaken your immune system.

Alcohol and Caffeine: Consume alcohol and caffeine in moderation. Excessive intake can interfere with sleep and potentially weaken your immune system.

Additional Considerations:

Food Sensitivities: Some individuals with herpes experience outbreak triggers related to certain foods. Identifying and avoiding these food triggers can be helpful. This may involve consulting a doctor or registered dietitian for personalized guidance.

Supplements: While there's no evidence to suggest any specific supplement can cure herpes, some may offer immune-boosting benefits. Discuss any supplements you're considering with your doctor to ensure they don't interact with your medications.

Exercise: Moving Your Body for Overall Health

Regular physical activity is essential for maintaining a healthy immune system. Here's why exercise should be part of your herpes management plan:

Boosts Immune System: Exercise promotes the production of white blood cells, the body's soldiers in fighting off infections.

Reduces Stress: Physical activity is a well-known stress reliever. As stress can trigger outbreaks, regular exercise can potentially reduce their frequency.

Improves Mood: Exercise releases endorphins, hormones that elevate mood and promote feelings of well-being. This can be particularly helpful during herpes outbreaks when you might be feeling low.

Finding Your Exercise Fit:

Choose Activities You Enjoy: The key to sticking with an exercise routine is finding activities you find enjoyable. This could be anything from brisk walking, swimming, cycling, dancing, or team sports.

Start Gradually: If you're new to exercise, start with short, low-intensity workouts and gradually increase the duration and intensity as your fitness improves.

Consistency is Key: Aim for at least 30 minutes of moderate-intensity exercise most days of the week. Consistency is more important than intensity.

Listen to Your Body:

Rest When Needed: During herpes outbreaks, you may need to modify your exercise routine or take rest days. Listen to your body and adjust your activity level accordingly.

Stress Management: Taming the Trigger

Stress can undeniably worsen herpes outbreaks. Here are some strategies to manage stress and potentially reduce the frequency and severity of your outbreaks:

Identify Stressors: The first step to managing stress is pinpointing what triggers your stress response. This could be work-related pressure, relationship issues, financial worries, or even a lack of sleep.

Relaxation Techniques: Practice relaxation techniques like yoga, meditation, deep breathing exercises, or progressive muscle relaxation.

Mindfulness: Mindfulness practices like meditation can help you become more aware of your thoughts and feelings and learn to respond to stress in a healthy way.

Support System: Having a strong support system of friends, family, or a therapist can provide a listening ear and emotional support during stressful times.

Sleep: The Foundation for Healing

Getting enough quality sleep is vital for overall health and immune function. Here's how prioritizing sleep can benefit your herpes management:

Cellular Repair: Sleep allows your body to repair and regenerate tissues, crucial during herpes outbreaks when healing is essential.

Immune System Function: Sleep deprivation can weaken your immune system, making you more susceptible to outbreaks.

MANAGING OUTBREAKS AND REDUCING FLARE-UPS

Herpes outbreaks, while unpredictable, can be managed effectively. This section delves into identifying potential triggers, understanding early warning signs, and implementing strategies to minimize outbreak severity and duration.

Understanding Your Triggers: Recognizing the Culprits

While the exact triggers for herpes outbreaks vary from person to person, some common culprits can exacerbate symptoms. Here's what to watch out for:

Stress: As previously discussed, stress can significantly impact your immune system and potentially trigger outbreaks.

Illness: Any illness, even a common cold, can weaken your immune system, making you more susceptible to herpes outbreaks.

Menstruation: Hormonal fluctuations during a menstrual cycle can trigger outbreaks in some women with genital herpes.

Sun Exposure: Sunburns or excessive sun exposure can trigger outbreaks, particularly for oral herpes (HSV-1).

Friction: Friction from tight clothing or vigorous sexual activity can irritate the genital area and potentially trigger outbreaks.

Certain Foods: Some individuals experience outbreak triggers related to specific foods. Identifying and avoiding these can be helpful.

Identifying Your Triggers:

Track Your Outbreaks: Keeping a journal to track outbreaks, including any potential triggers you might have experienced before the outbreak (stressful event, illness, etc.) can help identify patterns.

Work with Your Doctor: Discuss your suspected triggers with your doctor. They can help you analyze your patterns and personalize a management plan.

Early Warning Signs: Catching it Before it Starts

Knowing the early warning signs of an impending outbreak can help you take proactive steps to minimize its severity and duration. Here are some signs to watch out for:

Tingling, itching, or burning sensation: This is a common early warning sign for both oral and genital herpes. The sensation typically occurs in the area where the future sores will erupt.

Tenderness or pain: The affected area may become tender or painful before the ظهور (zuhūr: appearance) of visible sores.

Swollen lymph nodes: You may experience swollen lymph nodes in the groin (genital herpes) or neck (oral herpes).

The Importance of Early Intervention:

Antiviral medications: Taking antiviral medications as soon as you experience early warning signs can significantly shorten the duration and severity of the outbreak.

Remember:

It's crucial to consult your doctor and discuss the most appropriate course of action for early intervention.

Minimizing Severity and Duration: Strategies for a Milder Outbreak

Once an outbreak occurs, here are some strategies that can help minimize its severity and duration:

Antiviral Therapy: Follow your doctor's instructions regarding antiviral medication dosage and duration to maximize their effectiveness.

Pain Management: Over-the-counter pain relievers like ibuprofen or acetaminophen can help manage discomfort associated with sores.

Sitz Baths: Soaking the genital area in warm water (sitz bath) for 10-15 minutes several times a day can provide soothing relief and promote healing.

Loose-fitting Clothing: Wear loose-fitting, breathable cotton clothing to minimize irritation in the affected area.

Maintain Hygiene: Keep the affected area clean and dry to prevent secondary infections.

Additional Tips:

Avoid touching the sores: Touching the sores can spread the virus to other parts of your body or other individuals. Wash your hands thoroughly if you do touch the sores.

Avoid sexual contact: Refrain from sexual activity during an outbreak to prevent transmission to your partner(s).

Self-Care During Outbreaks: Prioritizing Your Well-being

During an outbreak, prioritizing self-care is crucial for promoting healing and emotional well-being. Here are some tips:

Rest: Get plenty of sleep to allow your body to focus on healing.

Hydration: Stay well-hydrated by drinking plenty of fluids.

Healthy Diet: Eat a healthy diet rich in fruits, vegetables, and whole grains to support your immune system.

Stress Management: Practice relaxation techniques like meditation or deep breathing to manage stress and promote healing.

Remember:

Dealing with an outbreak can be frustrating and emotionally draining. Allow yourself time to process your emotions and seek support from friends, family, or a therapist if needed.

PART 3: COPING WITH STIGMA

THE EMOTIONAL IMPACT OF HERPES

Part 3: Coping with Stigma: Navigating the Emotional Landscape

A diagnosis of herpes can be accompanied by a wave of emotions like anxiety, depression, and even shame. This section delves into the emotional impact of herpes stigma, offers strategies for building resilience and self-esteem, and explores available mental health support resources.

The Emotional Impact of Herpes

Living with herpes can be emotionally challenging due to the social stigma often associated with STIs. Here's a closer look at some common emotional responses:

Anxiety: You may experience anxiety about future outbreaks, potential transmission to partners, or rejection.

Depression: Feeling isolated, ashamed, or hopeless due to the stigma can lead to depression.

Trauma: The diagnosis itself, or negative experiences related to disclosure, can feel traumatic.

Building Resilience and Self-Esteem

Empowering yourself with knowledge and developing coping mechanisms is crucial in overcoming the emotional challenges of herpes. Here are some strategies:

Challenge Negative Thoughts: Identify and challenge negative self-talk associated with your diagnosis.

Focus on Facts: Educate yourself about herpes and dispel myths. Knowing the facts can help combat anxiety and empower you to communicate effectively with partners.

Practice Self-Compassion: Be kind and compassionate towards yourself. Remember, herpes is a common condition, and you are not alone.

Focus on Your Strengths: Focus on your positive attributes and accomplishments to boost your self-esteem.

Build a Strong Support System: Surround yourself with supportive friends, family, or therapists who offer understanding and encouragement.

PERSONAL STORIES OF LIVING WITH HERPES

Hearing from others who have walked a similar path can be incredibly validating and inspiring. Real-life stories can help you navigate your emotions and offer perspectives from individuals living fulfilling lives with herpes. Here are some avenues to explore:

Online Resources: Look for online platforms or support groups where individuals share their experiences of living with herpes. Reading their stories can provide valuable insights and a sense of community.

Books and Articles: Several books and articles delve into personal stories of living with herpes. These can offer a relatable perspective and practical advice.

Remember: Sharing your story, whether with a trusted friend, therapist, or online support group, can be incredibly empowering.

Mental Health Support and Resources

If you're struggling to cope with the emotional impact of herpes, seeking professional mental health support can be highly beneficial. Here are some resources readily available:

Therapy and Counseling: Talking to a therapist can provide a safe space to process your emotions, develop coping mechanisms, and work through any trauma related to your diagnosis.

Support Groups: Connecting with support groups can put you in touch with others who understand your challenges. You can share experiences, offer mutual support, and gain valuable coping strategies. Many online platforms and local organizations offer herpes-specific support groups.

Here are some resources to get you started:

National Network to End Domestic Violence: https://nnedv.org/ (While not specific to herpes, this resource can be helpful for individuals experiencing emotional distress or manipulation in relationships)

The Herpes Support Society: https://www.ashasexualhealth.org/herpes-support-groups/

Remember:

Seeking mental health support is a sign of strength and self-care. There's no shame in asking for help.

Living with herpes doesn't have to define your mental well-being. With knowledge, self-compassion, and access to support resources, you can effectively navigate the emotional landscape and live a fulfilling life.

PART 4: RELATIONSHIPS AND DISCLOSURE

NAVIGATING INTIMACY WITH CONFIDENCE

A herpes diagnosis doesn't have to spell doom for your relationships or sex life. Open and honest communication with potential and existing partners is key to building healthy and fulfilling connections. This section delves into communication strategies and safe sex practices to navigate intimacy with confidence.

Communication Strategies: The Power of Honesty

Communicating openly and honestly with potential and existing partners about your herpes status is essential. Here are some tips for effective communication:

Timing: Choose a time for a private conversation when you can have a thoughtful discussion without distractions.

Start with Education: Briefly explain herpes, the different types (HSV-1 and HSV-2), and the symptoms. Provide reliable sources like the Centers for Disease Control and Prevention (CDC) or Planned Parenthood websites for further information.

Focus on Facts: Reassure your partner that herpes is a common condition and doesn't define you.

Express Your Feelings: Share any anxieties or concerns you might have about disclosure.

Be Open to Questions: Encourage your partner to ask questions and address their concerns.

Respect Their Decision: Understand that your partner may need time to process the information.

Additional Tips:

Practice Disclosure: If talking about herpes feels overwhelming, practice what you'll say beforehand. Consider role-playing with a trusted friend or therapist.

Focus on Open Communication: Emphasize your commitment to open communication within the relationship and encourage your partner to share their sexual history and any potential concerns.

Remember:

Disclosure is an ongoing conversation. As your relationship progresses, you can discuss transmission risks, safe sex practices, and your individual needs related to herpes management.

Safe Sex Practices: Minimizing Transmission Risk

While herpes can be transmitted without visible sores (asymptomatic shedding), consistent and correct condom use can significantly reduce the risk. Here are some safe sex practices to consider:

Condoms: Using condoms every time you have sex, regardless of whether you have symptoms or not, significantly reduces the risk of transmission.

Correct Condom Use: Ensure you use condoms correctly and consistently for the entire duration of sexual activity.

Types of Condoms: Both latex and polyurethane condoms are effective for preventing herpes transmission.

Mutual Disclosure: Open communication about your herpes status allows your partner to make informed decisions regarding safe sex practices.

Additional Considerations:

Suppressive Therapy: If you're in a long-term, committed relationship, discuss suppressive therapy with your doctor. This can significantly reduce the risk of transmission to your partner even during periods of asymptomatic shedding.

Avoiding Sexual Activity During Outbreaks: Abstaining from sexual activity when you have visible sores is crucial to prevent transmission.

Oral Sex: While oral sex can transmit herpes, the risk is lower than genital-to-genital contact. Discuss safe sex practices with your partner, such as using dental dams, to further minimize risk.

Remember:

Safe sex practices are not just about preventing herpes transmission; they also protect against other sexually transmitted infections.

By prioritizing communication and safe sex practices, you can maintain healthy and fulfilling sexual relationships with herpes.

DISCLOSURE AND HONESTY

A herpes diagnosis can raise concerns about relationships and intimacy. However, open and honest communication is the cornerstone of building trust and maintaining healthy connections. This section delves deeper into the "when" and "how" of disclosure, offering strategies to build trust and support within your relationships.

When and How to Tell Partners: Finding the Right Moment

There's no one-size-fits-all answer to when you should disclose your herpes status to a partner. Here are some factors to consider:

Level of Intimacy: Consider the level of intimacy you've reached in the relationship. Disclosing before engaging in sexual activity is crucial, but the timing can be flexible depending on the situation.

Comfort Level: Choose a time when you feel comfortable and have the emotional space for a meaningful conversation.

Potential Partner's Readiness: If you're dating someone new, gauge their emotional readiness for potentially sensitive topics.

Tips for Disclosure:

Initiate the Conversation: Take the lead and initiate the conversation about your herpes status. Don't wait for your partner to bring it up.

Choose a Private Setting: Ensure you have a private space for a conversation without distractions.

Start with Education: Briefly explain herpes, the different types (HSV-1 and HSV-2), and the symptoms. Provide reliable sources like the Centers for Disease Control and Prevention (CDC) or Planned Parenthood websites for further information.

Focus on Facts: Reassure your partner that herpes is a common condition and doesn't define you.

Express Your Feelings: Share any anxieties or concerns you might have about disclosure.

Be Open to Questions: Encourage your partner to ask questions and address their concerns openly.

Remember:

There's no right or wrong script for disclosure. However, sincerity, honesty, and openness are key to fostering trust within your relationship.

Building Trust and Support: Fostering Connection

Open communication about your herpes status is the first step towards building trust and support within your relationships. Here's how to nurture understanding and connection:

Active Listening: Actively listen to your partner's concerns and questions about herpes. Be patient and allow them time to process the information.

Offer Resources: Share reliable resources like the American Sexual Health Association (ASHA) or Planned Parenthood websites that can provide your partner with further information about herpes.

Address Concerns: Be prepared to address your partner's concerns regarding transmission risk, safe sex practices, and potential impact on their health.

Focus on Shared Goals: Shift the conversation to finding solutions and fostering a supportive environment where you can navigate your relationship together.

Respect Decisions: Respect your partner's decision, whether they choose to continue the relationship or not.

Remember:

Building trust takes time. Open and honest communication, along with a willingness to address concerns, can foster a supportive relationship despite an herpes diagnosis.

Existing Relationships and Disclosure: Navigating Change

If you've already been in a relationship for a while before receiving a herpes diagnosis, disclosure can feel particularly challenging. Here's how to approach this situation:

Honesty is Key: While the timing of disclosure may not have been ideal, honesty remains vital. Explain your diagnosis and the reasons for not disclosing it earlier.

Reassurance and Support: Reassure your partner that you haven't intentionally put their health at risk and offer to answer any questions they might have.

Transparency: Be transparent about your steps towards managing your herpes with medication and safe sex practices.

Strengthen Communication: This might be a good time to revisit communication patterns within your relationship and emphasize the importance of open dialogue.

Remember:

While navigating disclosure in an existing relationship can be difficult, honesty and open communication can provide the foundation for rebuilding trust and moving forward together.

Finding Support Beyond Your Partner:

While your partner's support is crucial, you might also benefit from seeking support from additional sources:

Therapist: Consider individual or couple's therapy to address any anxieties or challenges related to your herpes diagnosis and its impact on your relationship.

Support Groups: Connecting with herpes-positive support groups can offer a sense of community, understanding, and practical tips for navigating relationships.

Remember:

You're not alone. Millions of people navigate fulfilling relationships with herpes. With open communication and a supportive network, you can build strong, healthy connections.

PHYSICAL SELF-CARE

Living with herpes requires a commitment to self-care that prioritizes both your physical and emotional well-being. This section delves into essential self-care practices, focusing on skincare and wound care during outbreaks, and exploring effective pain management strategies.

Physical Self-Care: Nurturing Your Body

Taking care of your physical health is crucial for managing herpes outbreaks and promoting overall well-being. Here are some key areas to focus on:

Healthy Diet: A balanced diet rich in fruits, vegetables, and whole grains provides your body with the essential nutrients needed to fight off infections and promote healing during outbreaks.

Regular Exercise: Regular physical activity strengthens your immune system, potentially reducing the frequency and severity of outbreaks. Choose activities you enjoy, like brisk walking, swimming, or dancing, and aim for at least 30 minutes of moderate-intensity exercise most days of the week.

Adequate Sleep: Prioritize getting enough quality sleep (7-8 hours per night) to allow your body to repair and regenerate tissues, crucial for healing during outbreaks.

Stress Management: Stress can be a trigger for outbreaks. Practice relaxation techniques like yoga, meditation, or deep breathing exercises to manage stress and promote overall well-being.

Skincare and Wound Care During Outbreaks

When you experience an outbreak, proper skincare and wound care can minimize discomfort and promote healing. Here's what to keep in mind:

Gentle Cleansing: Cleanse the affected area with warm water and a mild, fragrance-free cleanser. Avoid harsh scrubbing or rubbing, which can irritate the sores. Pat the area dry with a clean, soft towel.

Keep it Dry: Moisture can prolong healing. Allow the sores to air dry as much as possible. If necessary, dab the area gently with a clean cloth to absorb excess moisture.

Loose-fitting Clothing: Wear loose-fitting, breathable cotton clothing that allows air circulation to the affected area. Tight clothing can irritate the sores and slow healing.

Pain Relief: Over-the-counter pain relievers like ibuprofen or acetaminophen can help manage discomfort associated with the sores. Topical pain relievers like lidocaine cream may also offer temporary relief.

Additional Tips:

Avoid Irritation: Avoid harsh soaps, detergents, and other products that may irritate the sores.

Don't Touch or Burst the Sores: Touching or bursting the sores can increase the risk of infection and scarring.

Sitz Baths: Soaking the genital area in warm water (sitz bath) for 10-15 minutes several times a day can provide soothing relief and promote healing.

Remember:

If you experience any unusual symptoms during an outbreak, such as fever, severe pain, or swollen lymph nodes, consult your doctor to rule out any secondary infections.

Pain Management Strategies: Finding Relief During Outbreaks

Outbreaks can be painful. Here are some strategies to manage the discomfort:

Over-the-counter Pain Relievers: As mentioned earlier, over-the-counter pain relievers like ibuprofen or acetaminophen can help alleviate pain.

Topical Pain Relievers: Topical pain relievers like lidocaine cream can numb the area and provide temporary relief.

Warm Compresses: Applying warm compresses to the affected area can help soothe pain and promote healing.

Sitz Baths: As previously discussed, sitz baths can provide pain relief and promote healing during outbreaks.

Complementary Therapies:

Some individuals find relief with complementary therapies like:

Acupuncture: Acupuncture may offer pain relief by stimulating the release of endorphins, the body's natural pain relievers.

Massage Therapy: Massage therapy can promote relaxation and potentially reduce pain associated with outbreaks.

Remember:

If over-the-counter pain relievers and home remedies don't provide adequate relief, consult your doctor to discuss alternative pain management strategies or prescription medications.

By prioritizing physical self-care, proper skincare and wound care during outbreaks, and implementing effective pain management strategies, you can minimize discomfort and promote healing, allowing you to navigate outbreaks with greater ease.

EMOTIONAL SELF-CARE

Emotional Self-Care

Living with herpes requires a holistic approach to self-care that addresses not just physical health but also emotional well-being. Here, we delve into emotional self-care practices, focusing on mindfulness and meditation, and explore the benefits of creative expression.

Mindfulness and Meditation: Cultivating Inner Peace

A herpes diagnosis can trigger anxiety, stress, or even depression. Mindfulness and meditation practices can be powerful tools for managing difficult emotions and promoting inner peace.

Mindfulness: Mindfulness is the practice of paying attention to the present moment without judgment. It involves focusing on your thoughts, feelings, and bodily sensations in a non-reactive way. Mindfulness can help you become more aware of your emotional triggers and develop healthy coping mechanisms.

Meditation: Meditation is a form of mindfulness training that involves focusing your attention on a particular object, thought, or sensation. Regular meditation practice can cultivate calmness, improve focus, and reduce stress.

Benefits of Mindfulness and Meditation:

Stress Reduction: Mindfulness and meditation can help manage stress, a potential trigger for herpes outbreaks.

Improved Emotional Regulation: These practices can enhance your ability to manage difficult emotions and respond to challenges in a healthy way.

Increased Self-Awareness: Mindfulness can cultivate greater self-awareness, allowing you to identify your emotional triggers and develop coping mechanisms.

Getting Started with Mindfulness and Meditation:

There are numerous resources available to help you learn mindfulness and meditation techniques:

Guided Meditations: Many online platforms and apps offer guided meditations for beginners.

Meditation Classes: Consider joining a local meditation class or workshop to learn proper techniques and receive support.

Mindfulness Apps: Explore mindfulness apps that offer guided meditations and exercises to cultivate present-moment awareness.

Remember:

Mastering mindfulness and meditation takes time and practice. Be patient with yourself and focus on building a consistent practice routine.

Creative Expression and Self-Expression: Finding Your Voice

Creative expression offers a powerful outlet for processing emotions and promoting self-discovery.

Art Therapy: Explore art therapy, where you create art to express your emotions and explore inner experiences. Art therapy can be particularly helpful after a herpes diagnosis when you might be grappling with difficult feelings.

Journaling: Journaling allows you to express your thoughts and emotions freely. Writing about your experiences with herpes can be a cathartic experience and help you process any negative emotions.

Music: Playing or listening to music can be a powerful tool for managing stress and expressing emotions.

Benefits of Creative Expression:

Emotional Release: Creative expression allows you to release pent-up emotions and navigate challenging feelings in a healthy way.

Stress Reduction: Engaging in creative activities can promote relaxation and reduce stress levels.

Self-Discovery: Creative exploration can help you gain a deeper understanding of your thoughts and emotions.

Finding Your Creative Outlet:

There are no limitations when it comes to creative expression. Explore various avenues to see what resonates with you:

Writing: Try writing poetry, short stories, or journaling about your experiences.

Painting, Drawing, or Sculpting: Visual arts can be a powerful way to express yourself non-verbally.

Music: Playing an instrument, singing, or even just listening to music can be therapeutic.

Dance: Moving your body can be a great way to express yourself and release emotions.

Remember:

There's no right or wrong way to be creative. Explore different activities and find what brings you a sense of enjoyment and emotional release.

By incorporating emotional self-care practices like mindfulness, meditation, and creative expression into your routine, you can foster inner peace, manage difficult emotions, and build resilience in the face of a herpes diagnosis.

CONCLUSION

LIVING A FULFILLING LIFE WITH HERPES

Empowerment and Advocacy

A herpes diagnosis doesn't define you or limit your potential for a happy, fulfilling life. This concluding section empowers you to embrace self-acceptance, navigate relationships with confidence, and potentially become an advocate for herpes awareness.

Empowerment and Self-Acceptance

Living with herpes is a journey of self-acceptance and empowerment. Here are some key takeaways to embrace:

Herpes is Common: Millions of people worldwide have herpes, making it a common condition. You are not alone.

Knowledge is Power: Educate yourself about herpes, transmission risks, and management strategies. Knowledge empowers you to make informed decisions about your health and relationships.

Focus on Self-Care: Prioritizing self-care, both physically and emotionally, is crucial for your well-being and managing outbreaks effectively.

Challenge Negative Self-Talk: Replace negative thoughts about yourself with positive affirmations. Celebrate your strengths and accomplishments.

Embrace Your Voice: Open communication and self-advocacy are essential in fostering healthy relationships and navigating potential challenges.

Remember:

You have the power to navigate your life with herpes with confidence and self-compassion. Surround yourself with supportive people and prioritize activities that bring you joy.

Building Healthy Relationships: Communication and Trust

Open and honest communication is the cornerstone of building and maintaining healthy relationships with herpes.

Communicate Effectively: Talk to your partners openly and honestly about your herpes status. Share reliable resources and address any concerns they may have.

Practice Safe Sex: Consistent and correct condom use significantly reduces the risk of transmission. Explore additional safe sex practices like suppressive therapy if you're in a long-term relationship.

Respect Decisions: Respect your partner's choices, whether they choose to continue the relationship or not.

Remember:

Building healthy relationships requires trust and understanding. By prioritizing communication and safe sex practices, you can navigate your relationships with confidence.

Advocacy for Awareness: Making a Difference

If you feel empowered to do so, consider becoming an advocate for herpes awareness. Here are some ways you can contribute:

Share Your Story: Sharing your story, anonymously or publicly, can help break down stigma and empower others.

Support Awareness Campaigns: Support organizations raising awareness about herpes and advocating for research towards a cure.

Educate Your Community: Talk to friends, family, and acquaintances about herpes to dispel myths and promote understanding.

Benefits of Advocacy:

Empowering Others: By sharing your story and experiences, you can empower others living with herpes to embrace self-acceptance and navigate their diagnosis confidently.

Breaking Stigma: Advocacy helps break down the social stigma associated with herpes and promote understanding.

Supporting Research: Increased awareness can lead to increased resources and funding for research towards a cure or improved management strategies.

Remember:

Your voice matters. By becoming an advocate for herpes awareness, you can make a positive impact on the lives of others living with this condition.

Living a Fulfilling Life with Herpes: A Final Note

A herpes diagnosis may come with challenges, but it doesn't have to limit your potential for a happy and fulfilling life. With knowledge, self-care, and open communication, you can manage your symptoms effectively and build healthy relationships. Remember, you are not alone. Millions of people navigate fulfilling lives with herpes. Embrace self-acceptance, prioritize your well-being, and consider becoming an advocate for awareness. Together, we can break down stigma and create a more informed and supportive environment for everyone living with herpes.

RESOURCES FOR FURTHER SUPPORT

By prioritizing self-care, open communication, and embracing self-acceptance, you can manage your condition effectively and live a fulfilling life. This concluding section offers valuable resources for further support and information.

Living Well with Herpes: A Journey of Empowerment

Here are some key takeaways to empower yourself as you navigate life with herpes:

Herpes is Common: Millions of people worldwide have herpes, making it a common condition. You are not alone.

Knowledge is Power: Educate yourself about herpes, transmission risks, and management strategies. Knowledge empowers you to make informed decisions about your health and relationships.

Focus on Self-Care: Prioritizing self-care, both physically and emotionally, is crucial for your well-being and managing outbreaks effectively.

Challenge Negative Self-Talk: Replace negative thoughts about yourself with positive affirmations. Celebrate your strengths and accomplishments.

Embrace Your Voice: Open communication and self-advocacy are essential in fostering healthy relationships and navigating potential challenges.

Seek Support: Don't hesitate to seek support from healthcare professionals, therapists, or support groups to address any emotional challenges.

Remember:

You have the power to navigate your life with herpes with confidence and self-compassion. Surround yourself with supportive people and prioritize activities that bring you joy.

Building Healthy Relationships: Communication and Trust

Open and honest communication is the cornerstone of building and maintaining healthy relationships with herpes.

Communicate Effectively: Talk to your partners openly and honestly about your herpes status. Share reliable resources and address any concerns they may have.

Practice Safe Sex: Consistent and correct condom use significantly reduces the risk of transmission. Explore additional safe sex practices like suppressive therapy if you're in a long-term relationship.

Respect Decisions: Respect your partner's choices, whether they choose to continue the relationship or not.

Remember:

Building healthy relationships requires trust and understanding. By prioritizing communication and safe sex practices, you can navigate your relationships with confidence.

Resources for Further Support: A Network of Knowledge and Care

Living with herpes doesn't mean going it alone. Here's a compilation of valuable resources you can access for further support and information:

National Institutes of Health (NIH): The NIH website offers comprehensive information on herpes, including symptoms, diagnosis, treatment options, and clinical trials. [https://www.ncbi.nlm.nih.gov/books/NBK554

427/]](https://www.ncbi.nlm.nih.gov/books/NBK554427/)

Centers for Disease Control and Prevention (CDC): The CDC provides reliable information on STIs, including herpes, focusing on transmission risks, prevention strategies, and available resources.
https://npin.cdc.gov/pages/herpes-basics

Planned Parenthood: Planned Parenthood offers information on herpes, including symptoms, testing, treatment options, and resources for finding a sexual health clinic.
[https://www.plannedparenthood.org/blog/how-do-i-get-genital-herpes-treatment-and-what-is-it](https://www.plannedparenthood.org/blog/h

ow-do-i-get-genital-herpes-treatment-and-
what-is-it)

American Sexual Health Association (ASHA):
ASHA offers information on herpes, including
support groups, educational materials, and
resources for healthcare professionals.
[https://www.ashasexualhealth.org/](https://w
ww.ashasexualhealth.org/)

The Herpes Support Society: This non-profit
organization provides support groups,
educational materials, and resources for people
living with herpes.
[https://www.ashasexualhealth.org/herpes-
support-
groups/](https://www.ashasexualhealth.org/he
rpes-support-groups/)

Support Groups:

Connecting with others who understand the challenges of living with herpes can be immensely beneficial. Online and in-person support groups offer a safe space to share experiences, ask questions, and gain emotional support. Resources like The Herpes Support Society and online platforms can help you find support groups near you.

Mental Health Support:

If you're struggling to cope emotionally with your herpes diagnosis, consider seeking professional help from a therapist or counselor. Therapy can provide a safe space to process your emotions, develop coping mechanisms, and address any underlying challenges related to self-esteem or body image.

Remember:

There's no shame in seeking help. Many resources are available to support you on your journey with herpes.

Living a Fulfilling Life with Herpes: A Message of Hope

A herpes diagnosis doesn't have to limit your potential for a happy and fulfilling life. With knowledge, self-care, open communication, and the support of valuable resources, you can effectively manage your symptoms, build trusting relationships, and achieve your goals. Embrace self-acceptance, prioritize your well-being, and empower yourself to create a fulfilling life. Remember, you are not alone!!!